Anti-Inflammatory Diet Cookbook for Beginners

The Complete Culinary Guide to Reducing Inflammation and Healing Immune System for Whole Body Wellness with Easy, Delicious and Healthy Recipes

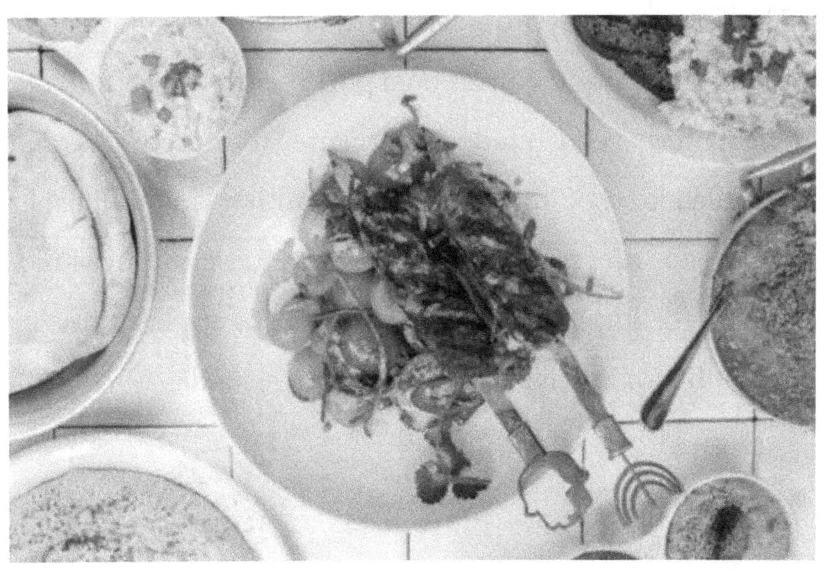

Tyrese Murray

Copyright © 2023 by Tyrese Murray

The information provided in this book is for general informational and educational purposes only. While every effort has been made to ensure the accuracy and completeness of the content, the author and publisher make no representations or warranties of any kind, express or implied, about the suitability, applicability, or reliability of the tips or guidelines presented.

CONTENTS

Dedication

This cookbook is dedicated to those who seek healing, promote wellbeing, and believe in the power of food as medicine. In a society dominated by processed meals and stressful lifestyles, your dedication to treating your body and spirit via mindful eating is extremely encouraging.

We dedicate "Anti-Inflammatory Diet Cookbook for Beginners" to those who are ready to take charge of their health and go on a journey to reduce inflammation, increase immunity, and achieve whole-body wellness. Your determination to prioritize healthful and pleasurable meals illustrates your resilience in the face of adversity.

May the recipes within these pages serve as a source of hope and direction on your path to flourishing health. From healthy breakfasts to satisfying dinners, each meal has been crafted with care to assist your body's natural healing processes while also infusing your taste buds with flavor and delight.

As you explore the culinary delights of the anti-inflammatory diet, may you find the deep impact that simple, nutritious ingredients can have on your well-being and vitality. May this cookbook be your valued companion as you journey toward wellness, providing inspiration, and practical idea for living a vibrant lifestyle.

With love and thanks.

Tyrese Murray

About the Author

Tyrese Murray is a renowned health and fitness instructor whose passion for transforming living has inspired many others on their paths to optimal wellness. Tyrese has become a trusted adviser for individuals seeking long-term lifestyle improvements because to his breadth of expertise in diet, fitness, and holistic health.

Tyrese, a trained fitness instructor and nutrition specialist, combines scientific knowledge with practical ways to make the sometimes difficult realm of health accessible to everyone. His dedication to empowering people is apparent in his coaching, writing, and public speaking careers.

Tyrese encourages individuals to unleash their potential with entertaining material and individualized coaching, emphasizing that health is a dynamic and joyful journey rather than a destination.

Tyrese Murray, who is on a quest to demystify the complexities of wellness, is a source of inspiration for individuals seeking long-term health breakthroughs. His work reflects the concept that everyone has the ability to design their own happiness, and Tyrese stays dedicated to leading people toward a life of energy and purpose.

Introduction

Welcome to a revolutionary culinary experience with the "Anti-Inflammatory Diet Cookbook for Beginners: The Complete Culinary Guide to Reducing Inflammation and Healing the Immune System for Whole Body Wellness with Easy, Delicious, and Healthy Recipes." In an age when the importance of diet on our health is becoming more widely recognized, this cookbook serves as a lighthouse for people seeking a holistic approach to health.

Inflammation, which is frequently the core cause of a variety of health problems, may be efficiently managed via the power of the foods we eat. This cookbook will guide you on your quest to reduce inflammation and rejuvenate your immune system for overall well-being.

Discover the secrets of an anti-inflammatory lifestyle as we walk you through the foundations of this transforming diet. Our recipes are designed for beginners, with an emphasis on simplicity and taste, to make adopting an anti-inflammatory diet a pleasurable and sustainable part of your daily life.

Immerse yourself in the pages of this culinary book, where each recipe is designed not just for taste, but also for its ability to treat inflammation and assist your body's natural healing mechanisms. This cookbook covers everything from nutrient-dense breakfasts to satisfying main dishes, delectable salads to guilt-free desserts, ensuring that your anti-inflammatory journey is not only healthy but also enjoyable.

Learn the fundamentals of an anti-inflammatory diet, the effects of chronic inflammation on your immune system, and the relationship between your food choices and general health. We'll walk you through setting up a beginner-friendly kitchen, adopting an anti-inflammatory lifestyle, and designing meal plans that are both simple to follow and nutritious.

Say goodbye to restricted diets and hello to a thriving, whole-body wellness experience. This "Anti-Inflammatory Diet Cookbook for Beginners" is more than simply a collection of recipes; it's an invitation to a healthier, more vibrant lifestyle. Join us on this flavorful adventure, where each bite helps to reduce inflammation, repair your immune system, and embrace a life of long-term well-being.

CHAPTER 1: UNDERSTANDING INFLAMMATION

Inflammation, often known as the body's natural response to damage or infection, is a complicated biological process that is essential for preserving health. This complicated process consists of a succession of immune responses designed to eliminate toxic stimuli, initiate tissue repair, and restore normal function. Understanding inflammation is critical for general well-being since it has a role in both acute and chronic health issues.

DEFINITION AND TYPES OF INFLAMMATION

In its most basic form, inflammation is the body's defense system against damaging stimuli. It manifests as a coordinated response that includes immune cells, blood vessels, and molecular mediators. The classic indications of inflammation—redness, swelling, heat, and pain—represent the body's attempt to cure itself. There are two main forms of inflammation:

Acute inflammation: This is the body's initial and rapid response to an injury or illness. It is a strictly controlled process that aims to eliminate the source of cell injury, remove damaged cells and tissues, and commence tissue healing. Acute inflammation usually lasts for a short time and then heals.

Chronic inflammation: On the other hand, is a long-term inflammatory response that can last weeks, months, or even years. Chronic inflammation, unlike acute inflammation, does not always resolve and can contribute to the advancement of a variety of illnesses, including autoimmune disorders and metabolic problems.

IMPACT OF CHRONIC INFLAMMATION ON THE IMMUNE SYSTEM

Acute inflammation is an essential and protective reaction, but prolonged inflammation can harm the immune system. Prolonged stimulation of inflammatory pathways can cause immune system dysregulation, in which the body's defensive mechanisms start attacking healthy tissues. This imbalance is linked to the development and worsening of autoimmune illnesses, in which the immune system erroneously attacks the body's cells.

Furthermore, chronic inflammation has been related to an elevated risk of a variety of health problems, including cardiovascular disease, diabetes, neurological disorders, and several malignancies. In this condition, the immune system is constantly activated, resulting in the production of pro-inflammatory chemicals that can cause tissue damage and malfunction.

CONNECTION BETWEEN DIET AND INFLAMMATION

Dietary choices have a dramatic impact on the control of inflammation in the body. Foods can either exacerbate or suppress the inflammatory process. Diets high in processed foods, sweets, and unhealthy fats have been linked to increased inflammation, which contributes to the development of chronic illnesses.

An anti-inflammatory diet, which includes whole foods, fruits, vegetables, fatty fish, nuts, and seeds, has been demonstrated to reduce inflammation and promote general health. The link between diet and inflammation emphasizes the need of adopting educated dietary decisions in order to ensure a healthy and harmonious immune response.

To summarize, a thorough grasp of inflammation is essential for everyone looking to improve their health. Recognizing the different types of inflammation, comprehending the impact of chronic inflammation on the immune system, and grasping the complex relationship between diet and inflammation enables people to make informed lifestyle decisions that promote general well-being and longevity.

Chapter 2: Basics of an Anti-Inflammatory Diet

Adopting an anti-inflammatory diet is a proactive and empowered way to improve overall health and well-being. This dietary strategy, based on the premise of eating foods that reduce inflammation, has grown in popularity due to its ability to reduce the risk of chronic illnesses and promote the body's natural healing processes.

List of Anti-Inflammatory Foods

The inclusion of foods with anti-inflammatory characteristics is an important component of an anti-inflammatory diet. This includes:

Fruits and vegetables: Fruits and vegetables are high in vitamins, minerals, fiber, and antioxidants, making them the cornerstone of any anti-inflammatory diet. Berries, leafy greens, citrus fruits, and cruciferous vegetables are well known for their anti-inflammatory properties.

Fatty Fish: Omega-3 fatty acids contained in fatty fish such as salmon, mackerel, and sardines have strong anti-inflammatory properties. These important fatty acids regulate the body's inflammatory response and contribute to overall cardiovascular health.

Nuts and seeds: Almonds, walnuts, flaxseed, and chia seeds are high in omega-3 fatty acids and antioxidants. These nuts and seeds may be easily incorporated into a variety of meals, adding both texture and nutritional content.

Whole Grains: Choosing whole grains over refined grains delivers vital minerals and fiber, which help to moderate the inflammatory response. Quinoa, brown rice, and oats are also healthful options in this category.

Healthy Fats: Olive oil, avocados, and almonds contain monounsaturated fats, which are anti-inflammatory. These fats promote heart health and general well-being.

Spices and herbs: Turmeric, ginger, garlic, and cinnamon are recognized for their anti-inflammatory and antioxidant effects. Incorporating these tasty items into your cooking not only improves the taste but also increases the nutritional value of your meals.

Anti-Inflammatory Foods to Eat:

Berries:

- Blueberries
- Strawberries
- Raspberries
- Blackberries
- Cherries

Leafy Greens:

- Spinach
- Kale
- Swiss chard
- Collard greens
- Arugula

Fatty Fish:

- Salmon
- Mackerel
- Sardines
- Trout
- Herring

Nuts and Seeds:

- Almonds
- Walnuts
- Flaxseeds
- Chia seeds
- Sunflower seeds

Whole Grains:

- Quinoa
- Brown rice
- Oats
- Barley
- Farro

Healthy Fats:

- Olive oil

- Avocado

- Nuts (especially almonds)

- Seeds (especially flaxseeds)

- Fatty fish (salmon, mackerel)

Spices and Herbs:

- Turmeric

- Ginger

- Garlic

- Cinnamon

- Rosemary

Colorful Vegetables:

- Bell peppers

- Tomatoes

- Broccoli

- Carrots

- Sweet potatoes

Legumes:

- Chickpeas

- Lentils

- Black beans

- Kidney beans

- Edamame

Green Tea:

- Green tea

- Matcha tea

- White tea

- Herbal teas (such as chamomile)

- Rooibos tea

FOODS TO AVOID FOR REDUCING INFLAMMATION

It is also critical to avoid pro-inflammatory foods when following an anti-inflammatory diet. Reducing or removing the following foods can help to achieve a more balanced inflammatory response:

Processed food: High in trans fats, refined carbohydrates, and additives, which can increase inflammation. Choose complete, unprocessed meals wherever feasible.

Sugary beverages: Soft drinks, juices, and energy drinks, can cause inflammation. Choosing water, herbal teas, or homemade fruit-infused water promotes hydration while minimizing inflammatory effects.

Red and processed meats: While lean meats may be part of a well-balanced diet, eating too much of them has been related to inflammation. Consider eating plant-based proteins such as beans, lentils, and tofu.

Excess Omega-6 Fatty Acids: While omega-6 fatty acids are necessary, an imbalance between omega-6 and omega-3 fatty acids can lead to inflammation. Reducing your intake of vegetable oils such as soybean and maize oil can aid in maintaining a better balance.

Refined grains: White bread and pasta, lack the fiber and minerals found in whole grains. Choosing whole grains over processed foods promotes an anti-inflammatory diet.

Pro-Inflammatory Foods to Avoid:

Processed Foods:

- Fast food items
- Packaged snacks (chips, crackers)
- Frozen meals
- Instant noodles
- Sugary cereals

Sugary Beverages:

- Soda
- Fruit-flavored drinks
- Energy drinks
- Sweetened iced tea
- Flavored coffee drinks

Red and Processed Meats:

- Bacon
- Sausages
- Hot dogs
- Processed deli meats
- Burgers high in saturated fat

Omega-6 Fatty Acids (Limit):

- Corn oil

- Soybean oil

- Safflower oil

- Sunflower oil

- Margarine

Refined Grains:

- White bread

- White rice

- Pastries and cakes

- Cookies

- White pasta

Dairy (Limit Full-Fat):

- Whole milk

- Full-fat yogurt

- Cheese

- Butter

- Cream

- Fried foods
- Commercially baked goods (cakes, pies)
- Margarine
- Microwave popcorn
- Some packaged snacks

Alcohol:

- Beer
- Wine
- Spirits
- Cocktails with added sugars
- Excessive consumption

Highly Processed Vegetable Oils:

- Cottonseed oil
- Palm oil
- Hydrogenated oils
- Vegetable shortening
- Industrial seed oils

Artificial Additives:

- Artificial sweeteners
- Artificial colors
- MSG (monosodium glutamate)
- High-fructose corn syrup
- Artificial preservatives

EXPLANATION OF THE ROLE OF ANTIOXIDANTS AND OMEGA-3 FATTY ACIDS

Antioxidants and omega-3 fatty acids are important in reducing inflammation and improving general health.

Antioxidants: Found plentiful in fruits, vegetables, and other plant-based meals, and they neutralize free radicals that cause inflammation and oxidative stress. Berries, dark leafy greens, and colorful vegetables have high levels of antioxidants, which help protect cells and tissues from harm.

Omega-3 Fatty Acids: These essential fatty acids, which are predominantly found in fatty fish, flaxseed, chia seeds, and walnuts, have anti-inflammatory properties. Omega-

3s are essential components of cell membranes, impacting both cellular function and immunological response. Incorporating these fats into your diet helps to maintain a balanced inflammatory state and improves heart health.

In conclusion, the fundamentals of an anti-inflammatory diet rely around mindful dietary choices that support a healthy equilibrium inside the body. The integration of anti-inflammatory foods, avoidance of pro-inflammatory choices, and recognizing the functions of antioxidants and omega-3 fatty acids all contribute to a comprehensive approach to promoting well-being and lowering inflammation. Individuals who embrace these dietary concepts can begin their road to maximum health and vigor.

Chapter 3: Getting Started with the Anti-Inflammatory Lifestyle

Adopting an anti-inflammatory lifestyle is a transforming journey that promotes general health and well-being. Making mindful decisions in your everyday life can greatly lower inflammation and help your body's natural healing processes. Let's look at the key factors of getting started with this life-changing method.

Tips for Transitioning to an Anti-Inflammatory Diet

Educate yourself.

Begin by learning the fundamentals of an anti-inflammatory diet. Discover which foods cause inflammation and which have anti-inflammatory effects. Knowledge is the foundation for making educated decisions.

Start gradually:

The transition to a new way of eating does not have to be sudden. Begin by making tiny modifications to your diet. Replace one pro-inflammatory item with an anti-inflammatory alternative, and gradually increase these changes.

Focus on Whole Foods:

Emphasize whole, unprocessed foods. Fresh fruits, vegetables, lean meats, and whole grains should be the foundation of your diet. Reduce your consumption of packaged and processed foods, which can include additives and preservatives.

Hydrate Mindfully:

Hydrate mindfully by choosing water, herbal teas, and other hydrating liquids. Sugary drinks should be reduced or eliminated, as they might lead to inflammation. Proper water promotes general health and helps to wash out pollutants.

Experiment with New Recipes:

Enjoy the change by trying new recipes. There are various delicious and gratifying recipes that support an anti-inflammatory lifestyle. Experimenting in the kitchen may transform your journey into a gourmet experience.

SETTING UP A BEGINNER-FRIENDLY KITCHEN

Stock up on Anti-Inflammatory Foods:

Ensure your kitchen has anti-inflammatory mainstays. Stock up on fruits, veggies, lean meats, nuts, seeds, and whole grains. Having these readily available makes dinner preparation easier.

Choose Healthy Cooking Oils:

Choose heart-healthy cooking oils, such as olive and avocado oil. These oils are high in monounsaturated fats, which add to the anti-inflammatory properties of your meals.

Invest in Quality Cookware:

Invest in high-quality cookware for a more pleasurable meal preparation experience. Consider investing in nonstick pans, stainless steel pots, and kitchen equipment that make cooking easier.

Eliminate pro-inflammatory culprits:

Eliminate or reduce pro-inflammatory substances from your cooking. This includes processed meals, sugary snacks, and omega-6-rich oils. Creating an atmosphere that supports your new lifestyle is critical.

Herbs and Spices Galore:

Enhance your cuisine with anti-inflammatory herbs and spices. Turmeric, ginger, garlic, cinnamon, and rosemary not only enhance the flavor of your dishes, but also increase their nutritious content.

Balance Macronutrients:

Balance Maintain a healthy balance of macronutrients in your meals, including carbs, proteins, and healthy fats. This balance encourages fullness while also providing your body with critical nutrients.

Include a Variety of Colors:

To create a bright platter, include a variety of fruits and vegetables. Different hues represent various phytonutrients, vitamins, and minerals that contribute to an anti-inflammatory diet.

Plan Ahead:

Plan your weekly meals ahead of time. This not only helps you organize your grocery list, but it also keeps you from making last-minute harmful food selections. Having a strategy in place prepares you for success.

Preparing in batches saves time and provides nutritional alternatives. Prepare greater quantities of grains, meats, and veggies to be utilized in several meals throughout the week.

Pay attention to your body's responses to different meals. Everyone is special, thus what works for one person may not work for another. Adjust your food plan to reflect how your body feels and behaves.

Finally, adopting an anti-inflammatory lifestyle is an empowering decision that leads to a healthier, more vibrant you. By implementing these principles, building a kitchen suited to your objectives, and developing a sustainable meal plan, you are embracing a lifestyle that promotes long-term well-being rather than merely a diet.

Chapter 4: Meal Planning and Preparation Tips

Effective meal planning and preparation are essential components of living a healthy lifestyle, particularly when following an anti-inflammatory diet. These practices not only save time, but they also enable people to make conscious decisions, ensuring that their meals adhere to the principles of lowering inflammation and improving general well-being.

Weekly Meal Plan Strategies

Set Realistic Goals:

Set achievable weekly goals. Consider your schedule, nutritional preferences, and the quantity of meals you'll need to prepare. Setting realistic goals makes the process more bearable.

Create a Weekly Menu:

Make a weekly meal with anti-inflammatory foods. Balance your meals with a variety of proteins, complete grains, healthy fats, and colorful fruits and veggies.

Check Inventory:

Before grocery shopping, check your pantry, refrigerator, and freezer. To reduce waste, take inventory of your current ingredients and plan meals around them.

Make a Detailed Shopping List:

Create a thorough shopping list based on your weekly meals. This reduces the likelihood of impulse purchases and ensures you have all of the materials on hand.

Prep Ingredients Ahead:

Prepare ingredients ahead of time by washing, cutting, and portioning them. Preparing materials ahead of time makes weekly cooking more effective.

Choose Batch-Friendly Recipes:

Choose recipes that suit batch cooking perfectly well. Soups, stews, casseroles, and grains are all great possibilities for large-scale cooking.

Invest in Storage Containers:

Invest in freezer-friendly storage containers. Divide batch-cooked dishes into individual servings for convenient thawing and reheating.

Label and Date:

Label containers with the dish name and date of preparation. This allows you to quickly identify and rotate your frozen meals while retaining freshness.

Utilize Freezer-Friendly Ingredients:

Use freezer-friendly foods such cooked grains, beans, and sauces. Prepare these elements in big amounts and freeze for later use.

Plan ahead of time to safely defrost frozen meals before consumption. Transfer the meal to the refrigerator the night before to ensure a safe and gradual defrost.

INCORPORATING ANTI-INFLAMMATORY PRINCIPLES INTO DAILY LIFE

Mindful Cooking Techniques:

Use mindful cooking procedures to retain the nutritional value of anti-inflammatory foods. Instead of frying, try steaming, sautéing, or baking.

Choose Whole Foods:

Choose complete, unprocessed meals wherever feasible. These foods are high in minerals and antioxidants, which contribute to the anti-inflammatory properties of your diet.

Experiment with Anti-Inflammatory Ingredients:

Explore various anti-inflammatory herbs and spices. Incorporate turmeric, ginger, garlic, and cinnamon into your recipes to boost taste while providing anti-inflammatory effects.

Hydrate Wisely:

Hydrate wisely by drinking water and herbal teas instead than sugary or caffeinated beverages. Proper hydration improves overall health and compliments an anti-inflammatory lifestyle.

Practice Portion Control:

To prevent overeating, practice portion control by paying attention to serving sizes. Consuming well-balanced and suitably proportioned meals helps to maintain stable blood sugar levels and promotes anti-inflammatory behaviour.

Finally, meal planning and preparation are crucial skills for anybody looking to adopt and maintain an anti-inflammatory lifestyle. By adopting these ideas into your daily routine, you may save time, decrease stress, and guarantee that your meals are regularly beneficial to your general health. Remember that these habits are more than simply what you eat; they are about developing a sustainable and health-conscious attitude to sustaining your body on a daily basis.

Chapter 5: Anti-Inflammatory Diet Sample Meal Plan

Day 1:

• Breakfast: Oatmeal with fresh berries and chia seeds.

• Lunch: Quinoa salad with mixed veggies, chickpeas, and lemon-tahini dressing.

• Dinner: Baked salmon, sweet potato wedges, and steamed broccoli.

• Snack on Greek yogurt with honey and nuts.

• Dessert: Baked apples with cinnamon.

Day 2:

• Breakfast: Smoothie with spinach, banana, blueberries, and almond milk.

• Lunch: Lentil soup with full grain crackers.

• Dinner: Grilled chicken breast, quinoa, and roasted Brussels sprouts.

• Snack: carrot and cucumber sticks together with hummus.

• Dessert: Mixed berry and coconut milk chia pudding.

Day 3:

• Breakfast: Greek yogurt parfait with granola, sliced strawberries, and honey.

• Lunch: Stuffed bell peppers with spinach and feta, served with mixed greens.

• Dinner: Turkey meatballs with zucchini noodles and tomato sauce.

• Snack: Apple slices and almond butter.

• Dessert: Mango Sorbet.

Day 4:

• Breakfast: Overnight oats with sliced peaches and maple syrup.

• Lunch: Quinoa and black bean dish with avocado, tomatoes, and cilantro.

• Dinner: Baked cod with quinoa and roasted asparagus.

• Snack: Mixed nuts and dried cranberries.

• Dessert: Baked pears with cinnamon.

Day 5:

• Breakfast: Whole grain toast together with avocado and cherry tomatoes.

• Lunch: Chickpea salad with cucumber, tomato, and lemon-herb dressing.

• Dinner: Grilled shrimp, brown rice, and sautéed spinach.

• Snack: Cottage cheese and pineapple chunks.

• Dessert: A berry and banana smoothie.

Day 6:

• Breakfast: Scrambled eggs with sautéed kale and whole-grain bread.

• Lunch: Mediterranean quinoa salad topped with olives, cherry tomatoes, and feta cheese.

• Dinner: Baked chicken breast, quinoa, and roasted sweet potatoes.

• Snack: Edamame with sea salt.

• Dessert: Coconut and berry frozen yogurt.

Day 7:

• Breakfast: Acai bowl with granola, banana slices, and shredded coconut.

• Lunch: Brown rice dish with blackened salmon, avocado, and mango salsa.

• Dinner: Stir-fried tofu, broccoli, and quinoa.

• Snack: Sliced cucumber with tzatziki sauce.

• Dessert: Dark chocolate-covered strawberries.

Day 8:

• Breakfast: Fruit smoothie with kale, pineapple, banana, and coconut water.

• Lunch: Lentil and vegetable curry together with basmati rice.

• Dinner: Grilled turkey burgers, sweet potato wedges, and green beans.

• Snack: Mixed berries and Greek yogurt.

• Dessert: Chia seed pudding with vanilla almond milk.

Day 9:

• Breakfast: Whole-grain English muffin with smashed avocado and poached eggs.

• Lunch: Quinoa and vegetable-stuffed acorn squash.

• Dinner: Baked fish with lemon and dill, paired with quinoa and steamed broccoli.

• Snack: sliced bell peppers with hummus.

• Dessert: Mango and coconut sorbet.

Day 10:

Breakfast: Overnight oats with sliced bananas and almond butter.

• Lunch: Chickpea and vegetable stir-fry over brown rice.

• Dinner: Grilled chicken skewers, quinoa, and roasted Brussels sprouts.

• Snack: Mixed nuts and dried apricots.

• Dessert: A berry and almond milk smoothie.

Day 11:

• Breakfast: Greek yogurt with granola, mixed berries, and honey.

• Lunch: Quinoa and black bean wrap with avocado, lettuce, and salsa.

• Dinner: Baked fish, quinoa, and roasted sweet potatoes.

• Snack: Carrot sticks and tzatziki sauce.

• Dessert: Baked apples with cinnamon.

Day 12:

• Breakfast: Acai smoothie with mixed berries and protein powder.

• Lunch: Chickpea and vegetable curry with basmati rice.

• Dinner: Grilled chicken breast, quinoa, and roasted sweet potatoes.

• Snack: Sliced apple and nut butter.

• Dessert: Chia seed pudding with vanilla almond milk.

Day 13:

• Breakfast: Acai smoothie bowl with oats, kiwi, and shredded coconut.

• Lunch: Lentil and vegetable soup with healthy grain crackers.

• Dinner: Turkey meatballs with whole grain spaghetti and tomato-basil sauce.

• Snack: Sliced cucumber with hummus.

• Dessert: Baked pears drizzled with honey.

• Breakfast: Whole grain toast together with avocado and cherry tomatoes.

• Lunch: Mediterranean quinoa salad topped with olives, cherry tomatoes, and feta cheese.

• Dinner: Grilled shrimp, brown rice, and sautéed spinach.

• Snack: Cottage cheese and pineapple chunks.

• Dessert: A berry and banana smoothie.

WEEK THREE

Day 15:

• Breakfast: Scrambled eggs with sautéed kale and whole-grain bread.

• Lunch: Chickpea salad with cucumber, tomato, and lemon-herb dressing.

• Dinner: Baked chicken breast, quinoa, and roasted sweet potatoes.

• Snack: Edamame with sea salt.

• Dessert: Coconut and berry frozen yogurt.

Day 16:

• Breakfast: Acai bowl with granola, banana slices, and shredded coconut.

• Lunch: Brown rice dish with blackened salmon, avocado, and mango salsa.

• Dinner: Stir-fried tofu, broccoli, and quinoa.

• Snack: Sliced cucumber with tzatziki sauce.

• Dessert: Dark chocolate-covered strawberries.

Day 17:

• Breakfast: Smoothie with kale, pineapple, banana, and coconut water.

• Lunch: Lentil and vegetable curry together with basmati rice.

• Dinner: Grilled turkey burgers, sweet potato wedges, and green beans.

- Snack: Mixed berries and Greek yogurt.

- Dessert: Chia seed pudding with vanilla almond milk.

Day 18:

- Breakfast: Whole-grain English muffin with smashed avocado and poached eggs.

- Lunch: Quinoa and vegetable-stuffed acorn squash.

- Dinner: Baked fish with lemon and dill, paired with quinoa and steamed broccoli.

- Snack: sliced bell peppers with hummus.

- Dessert: Mango and coconut sorbet.

Day 19:

Breakfast: Overnight oats with banana slices and almond butter.

- Lunch: Chickpea and vegetable stir-fry over brown rice.

- Dinner: Grilled chicken skewers, quinoa, and roasted Brussels sprouts.

- Snack: Mixed nuts and dried apricots.

• Dessert: A berry and almond milk smoothie.

• Breakfast: Greek yogurt with granola, mixed berries, and honey.

• Lunch: Quinoa and black bean wrap with avocado, lettuce, and salsa.

• Dinner: Baked fish, quinoa, and roasted sweet potatoes.

• Snack: Carrot sticks and tzatziki sauce.

• Dessert: Baked apples with cinnamon.

Day 21:

• Breakfast: Spinach and feta omelet with whole grain bread.

• Lunch: Kale and quinoa salad with roasted chickpeas, tomatoes, and balsamic vinaigrette.

• Dinner: Grilled shrimp with quinoa and veggie medley.

• Snack: Greek yogurt and sliced strawberries.

• Dessert: Mixed Berry Sorbet.

Day 22:

• Breakfast: Banana and almond butter smoothie.

• Lunch: Whole-grain pita with hummus, cucumber, and cherry tomatoes.

• Dinner: Baked chicken thighs, sweet potato wedges, and sautéed greens.

• Snack: Sliced apple and nut butter.

• Dessert: Avocado chocolate mousse.

Day 23:

• Breakfast: Quinoa porridge with mixed berries and honey.

• Lunch: Lentil and veggie wrap with tahini dressing.

• Dinner: Grilled tilapia with quinoa and steamed broccoli.

• Snack: Trail mix with nuts and dried fruits.

• Dessert: Mango and Coconut Chia Pudding.

Day 24:

• Breakfast: Whole-grain bread with ricotta cheese and sliced strawberries.

• Lunch: Greek salad with chickpeas, feta cheese, olives, and a lemon-olive oil vinaigrette.

• Dinner: Turkey and vegetable stir-fry over brown rice.

• Snack: Sliced cucumber with tzatziki sauce.

• Dessert: A mixed berry smoothie bowl.

Day 25:

• Breakfast consisted of scrambled eggs with sautéed spinach and cherry tomatoes.

• Lunch: Quinoa and black bean dish with avocado, salsa, and lime juice.

• Dinner: Baked fish with lemon-herb marinade, quinoa, and roasted Brussels sprouts.

• Snack: Greek yogurt and walnuts.

• Dessert: Dark chocolate-covered banana slices.

Day 26:

• Breakfast: Acai smoothie with mixed berries and protein powder.

• Lunch: Chickpea and vegetable curry with basmati rice.

• Dinner: Grilled chicken breast, quinoa, and roasted sweet potatoes.

• Snack: Sliced apple and nut butter.

• Dessert: Chia seed pudding with vanilla almond milk.

Day 27:

• Breakfast: Whole-grain English muffin with smashed avocado and poached eggs.

• Lunch: Quinoa and vegetable-stuffed bell peppers.

• Dinner: Baked salmon, quinoa, and steamed broccoli.

• Snack: Trail mix with nuts and dried fruits.

• Dessert: Avocado chocolate mousse.

Day 28:

• Breakfast: Greek yogurt with granola, mixed berries, and honey.

• Lunch: Lentil and vegetable soup with healthy grain crackers.

• Dinner: Grilled turkey burgers, quinoa, and roasted veggies.

• Snack: Sliced cucumber with hummus.

• Dessert: Mixed Berry Sorbet.

CHAPTER 6: HEALTHY ANTI-INFLAMMATORY DIET RECIPES

Turmeric Smoothie

This dynamic turmeric smoothie could be tasty and nutritious way to kickstart your day, giving a burst of anti-inflammatory goodness.

- **Preparation time**: 5 minutes
- **Cook Time**: 0 minutes
- **Servings**: 2

Ingredients:

- 1 glass Greek yogurt

- 1 glass solidified blended berries

- 1 ripe banana

- 1 teaspoon ground turmeric

- Sprint of black pepper

- Modest bunch of new spinach

- 1 container almond milk

- 1 Icecube (discretionary)

Instructions:

1. In a blender, combine Greek yogurt, solidified berries, banana, turmeric, black pepper, spinach, and almond milk.

2. Mix until smooth. In case wanted, include ice cubes and mix once more for a colder consistency.

3. Pour into glasses and serve quickly.

Nutritional Information: Per Serving (approx.):

- Calories: 250

- Protein: 15g

- Fat: 8g

- Carbohydrates: 35g

- Fiber: 7g

Notes:

• For included sweetness, you can incorporate a sprinkle of honey or a sprinkle of maple syrup.

Oatmeal with Berries and Nuts

A healthy and nutritious cereal bowl highlighting the anti-inflammatory benefits of oats, berries, and nuts.

- **Prep Time:** 5 minutes
- **Cook Time:** 10 minutes
- **Servings:** 2

Ingredients:

• 1 container old-fashioned oats

• 2 glasses of water or milk of choice

• 1 container blended berries (blueberries, strawberries)

• 1/4 container chopped walnuts or almonds

• Nectar or maple syrup (discretionary)

• Pinch of cinnamon (discretionary)

Instructions:

1. In a pan, bring oats and water or milk to a bubble. Reduce warm and simmer until oats are cooked, blending once in a while.

2. Separate cooked oats into bowls and top with mixed berries and chopped nuts.

3. Sprinkle with nectar or maple syrup and sprinkle with cinnamon in case wanted.

Nutritional Information: Per Serving (approx.):

- Calories: 300

- Protein: 10g

- Fat: 12g

- Carbohydrates: 40g

- Fiber: 7g

Notes:

- Feel free to customize along with your favorite natural products

Salmon and Avocado Toast

A savory and fulfilling breakfast highlighting the inflammation-fighting properties of omega-3 fatty acids in salmon and healthy fats in avocado.

- **Prep Time:** 10 minutes
- **Cook Time:** 5 minutes
- **Servings:** 2

Ingredients:

- 2 cuts whole-grain bread, toasted

- 1 ripe avocado, pounded

- 4 oz smoked salmon

- Lemon wedges for decorate

- Fresh dill (discretionary)

Instructions:

1. Toast the whole-grain bread cuts until golden brown.

2. Spread squashed avocado equitably on each cut.

3. Top with smoked salmon, a press of lemon juice, and embellish with fresh dill if wanted.

Nutritional Information: Per Serving (approx.):

• Calories: 320

• Protein: 18g

• Fat: 18g

• Carbohydrates: 25g

Notes:

• For additional flavor, squeeze of ocean salt and black pepper to the squashed avocado.

Chia Seed Pudding with Mango

A delightful chia seed pudding imbued with anti-inflammatory omega-3s and topped with sweet mango.

- **Prep Time:** 5 minutes (plus overnight chilling)
- **Cook Time:** 0 minutes
- **Servings:** 2

Ingredients:

- 1/4 glass chia seeds

- 1 glass almond milk

- 1 tablespoon nectar

- 1 teaspoon vanilla extract

- 1 diced ripe mango,

Instructions:

1. In a bowl, whisk together chia seeds, almond milk, nectar, and vanilla extract.

2. Cover and refrigerate overnight or for at slightest 4 hours, permitting the chia seeds to assimilate the fluid and shape a pudding-like consistency.

3. Spoon the chia pudding into serving bowls and top with diced mango.

Nutritional Information: Per Serving (approx.):

- Calories: 220

- Protein: 5g

- Fat: 10g

- Carbohydrates: 30g

- Fiber: 12g

Notes:

- Explore with diverse natural product fixings for assortment.

Greek Yogurt Parfait

A reviving and protein-packed Greek yogurt parfait filled with probiotics, cancer prevention agents, and anti-inflammatory supplements.

- **Prep Time:** 5 minutes
- **Cook Time:** 0 minutes
- **Servings:** 2

Ingredients:

- 1 glass Greek yogurt

- 1 cup freshly diced pineapple or papaya

- 2 tablespoons nectar

• 1/4 glass chopped nuts (almonds, pistachios)

Instructions:

1. In glasses or bowls, layer Greek yogurt with diced pineapple or papaya.

2. Sprinkle each layer with nectar and chopped nuts.

3. Rehash the layers until the glass is filled.

Nutritional Information: Per Serving (approx.):

• Calories: 280

• Protein: 15g

• Fat: 12g

• Carbohydrates: 30g

• Fiber: 3g

Notes:

• Select plain Greek yogurt to control added sugars, and customize together with your favorite natural products and nuts.

Egg and Spinach Breakfast Wrap

A nutritious and flavorful breakfast wrap including scrambled eggs, fresh spinach, tomatoes, and creamy avocado.

- **Prep Time:** 10 minutes
- **Cook Time:** 5 minutes
- **Servings:** 2

Ingredients:

- 4 whole-grain tortillas

- 6 eggs, scrambled

- 2 cups fresh spinach leaves

- 1 tomato, sliced

- 1 avocado, cut

Instructions:

1. Heat the whole-grain tortillas in a dry skillet until warm.

2. In a separate dish, scramble the eggs until completely cooked.

3. Assemble the wraps by putting scrambled eggs, new spinach, Sliced tomato , and avocado on each tortilla.

4. Roll up the tortillas into wraps and serve instantly.

Nutritional Information: (Per serving)

• Calories: 380

• Protein: 18g

• Carbohydrates: 35g

• Fat: 20g

• Fiber: 8g

Notes:

• Feel free to include a sprinkle of feta cheese or hot sauce for extra flavor.

Berry and Almond Butter Smoothie Bowl

A scrumptious and antioxidant-rich smoothie bowl with blended berries, almond butter, and nutritious seeds.

- **Prep Time:** 5 minutes
- **Servings:** 2

Ingredients:

- 2 glasses blended berries (blueberries, strawberries, raspberries)

- 2 tablespoons almond butter

- 1 glass almond milk

- 2 tablespoons chia seeds

- 2 tablespoons hemp seeds

Instructions:

1. Blend mixed berries, almond butter, and almond milk until smooth.

2. Pour the smoothie into bowls and top with chia seeds and hemp seeds.

Nutritional Information: (Per serving)

- Calories: 280

- Protein: 8g

- Carbohydrates: 30g

- Fat: 15g

- Fiber: 10g

Notes:

- Customize with your favorite toppings, such as granola or sliced banana.

Sweet Potato and Kale Breakfast Hash

A nutrient-dense breakfast hash including grated sweet potatoes, sautéed kale, and discretionary poached or fried egg.

Prep Time: 15 minutes

Cook Time: 15 minutes

Servings: 4

Ingredients:

- 2 big sweet potatoes, grated

- 2 cups kale, chopped

- 1 red onion, diced

- 2 tablespoons olive oil

- Salt and pepper to taste

- 4 poached or fried eggs (discretionary)

Instructions:

1. In a large pan, sauté grated sweet potatoes, chopped kale, and diced red onion in olive oil until cooked.

2.Flavor with salt and pepper as desired.

3. Alternatively, top each serving with a poached or fried egg.

Nutritional Information: (Per serving, without egg)

- Calories: 220

- Protein: 4g

- Carbohydrates: 40g

- Fat: 7g

- Fiber: 6g

Notes:

- Include a sprinkle of feta cheese or hot sauce for additional flavor.

Cottage Cheese and Pineapple Bowl

A refreshing and protein-packed breakfast bowl including cottage cheese, fresh pineapple, and crunchy nuts.

- **Prep Time:** 5 minutes
- **Servings:** 2

Ingredients:

- 2 cups cottage cheese

- 1 cup fresh pineapple chunks

- 1/4 cup walnuts or almonds, chopped

- Cinnamon for sprinkling (discretionary)

Instructions:

1. In bowls, layer cottage cheese, fresh pineapple chunks, and chopped nuts.

2. Alternatively, sprinkle with cinnamon for added flavor.

Nutritional Information: (Per serving)

- Calories: 280

- Protein: 28g

- Carbohydrates: 20g

- Fat: 10g

- Fiber: 2g

Notes:

- Select unsweetened cottage cheese for a healthier alternative.

Mushroom and Tomato Scramble

A savory and satisfying egg scramble with sautéed mushrooms, cherry tomatoes, and fresh basil.

- **Prep Time:** 10 minutes
- **Cook Time:** 10 minutes
- **Servings:** 2

Ingredients:

- 4 eggs, scrambled

- 2 cups mushrooms, cut

- 1 container cherry tomatoes, halved

- 2 tablespoons fresh basil, chopped

- 1 tablespoon olive oil

- Salt and pepper as desired

Instructions:

1. In a skillet, sauté sliced mushrooms in olive oil until golden.

2. Include scrambled eggs, cherry tomatoes, and fresh basil.

3. Cook until eggs are set and tomatoes are slightly softened.

4. Flavor with salt and pepper as desired.

Nutritional Information: (Per serving)

- Calories: 240

- Protein: 16g

- Carbohydrates: 8g

- Fat: 18g

- Fiber: 2g

Notes:

• Combine with whole-grain toast for a complete meal.

Grilled Chicken and Quinoa Salad

A light and nutritious salad including barbecued chicken, quinoa, and an assortment of fresh vegetables.

- **Prep Time:** 15 minutes
- **Cook Time**: 15 minutes
- **Servings**: 4

Ingredients:

• 4 barbecued chicken breasts

• 2 glasses cooked quinoa

• 4 glasses blended greens (kale, spinach)

• 1 glass cherry tomatoes, halved

• 1 cucumber, sliced

• 1 avocado, diced

- Olive oil and lemon dressing

Instructions:

1. In a big bowl, combine barbecued chicken, cooked quinoa, blended greens, cherry tomatoes, cucumber, and diced avocado.

2. Sprinkle with olive oil and lemon dressing and toss gently.

3. Serve instantly.

Nutritional Information: (Per serving)

- Calories: 400

- Protein: 30g

- Carbohydrates: 30g

- Fat: 20g

- Fiber: 8g

Notes:

• Feel free to customize the salad along with your favorite vegetables or include a sprinkle of feta cheese for additional flavor.

Vegetarian Lentil Stew

A hearty and filling vegetarian stew including lentils, sweet potatoes, and an array of colorful vegetables.

- **Prep Time:** 20 minutes
- **Cook Time:** 30 minutes
- **Servings:** 6

Ingredients:

• 2 glasses lentils, washed

• 2 sweet potatoes, diced

• 3 glasses infant spinach leaves

• 1 onion, diced

• 3 cloves garlic, minced

• 4 glasses vegetable broth

- 1 teaspoon turmeric

- 1 teaspoon cumin

- 1 teaspoon paprika

Instructions:

1. In a big pot, sauté onions and garlic until softened.

2. Include lentils, sweet potatoes, infant spinach, vegetable broth, turmeric, cumin, and paprika.

3. Simmer until lentils and sweet potatoes are tender.

4. Serve hot.

Nutritional Information: (Per serving)

- Calories: 350

- Protein: 18g

- Carbohydrates: 60g

- Fat: 2g

- Fiber: 15g

Notes:

• Garnish with fresh herbs like cilantro or parsley before serving.

Salmon and Broccoli Stir-Fry

A quick and flavorful stir-fry including salmon, broccoli, and vibrant vegetables.

- **Prep Time:** 15 minutes
- **Cook Time:** 10 minutes
- **Servings:** 4

Ingredients:

• 4 salmon fillets

• 2 glasses broccoli florets

• 1 bell pepper, sliced

• 1 cup snow peas

• 1 tablespoon ginger powder

• 3 tablespoons low-sodium soy sauce

Instructions:

1. In a pan, sauté salmon, broccoli, bell pepper, snow peas, and ginger powder until salmon is cooked through.

2. Sprinkle with low-sodium soy sauce and stir-fry for an extra 2 minutes.

3. Serve over brown rice if wanted.

Nutritional Information: (Per serving)

- Calories: 320

- Protein: 25g

- Carbohydrates: 15g

- Fat: 18g

- Fiber: 5g

Notes:

- Adjust soy sauce amount based on individual preference for saltiness.

Quinoa and Chickpea Buddha Bowl

A feeding and colorful Buddha bowl including quinoa, chickpeas, and dynamic vegetables.

- **Prep Time:** 15 minutes
- **Servings:** 3

Ingredients:

- 2 glasses cooked quinoa

- 1 can chickpeas, drained and washed

- 2 cups roasted sweet potatoes, cubed

- 1 avocado, sliced

- 1 container shredded red cabbage

- Tahini dressing

Instructions:

1. Arrange cooked quinoa, chickpeas, roasted sweet potatoes, avocado slices, and shredded red cabbage in a bowl.

2. Sprinkle with tahini dressing.

Nutritional Information: (Per serving)

- Calories: 420

- Protein: 15g

- Carbohydrates: 60g

- Fat: 15g

- Fiber: 12g

Notes:

- Include a sprinkle of sesame seeds for additional crunch.

Turkey and Vegetable Skewers with Tzatziki

Tasty and lean turkey skewers with a side of refreshing tzatziki sauce.

- **Prep Time:** 20 minutes
- **Cook Time:** 15 minutes
- **Servings:** 4

Ingredients:

- 1 pound turkey breast, cubed

- 1 glass cherry tomatoes

- 1 red onion, diced

- 2 bell peppers, cut

- 2 zucchinis, cut

- Tzatziki sauce for dipping

Instructions:

1. Thread turkey, cherry tomatoes, red onion, bell peppers, and zucchini onto skewers.

2. Barbecue or heat until turkey is cooked through.

3. Serve with a side of tzatziki sauce.

Nutritional Information: (Per serving)

- Calories: 280

- Protein: 30g

- Carbohydrates: 15g

- Fat: 10g

- Fiber: 5g

Notes:

• Marinate turkey in your favorite Mediterranean spices to enhanced flavor.

Mango and Shrimp Salad

A refreshing and tropical salad including shrimp, diced mango, and a zesty lime vinaigrette.

- **Prep Time:** 15 minutes
- **Cook Time:** 5 minutes
- **Servings:** 3

Ingredients:

• 1 pound shrimp, cooked

• 1 mango, diced

• 4 glasses blended greens (arugula, watercress)

• 1/2 red onion, thinly sliced

• 1/4 container of chopped cilantro

• Lime vinaigrette

Instructions:

1. Stir fry cooked shrimp, diced mango, mixed greens, thinly cut red onion, and chopped cilantro in a bowl.

2. Sprinkle with lime vinaigrette and mix well.

Nutritional Information: (Per serving)

- Calories: 220

- Protein: 25g

- Carbohydrates: 20g

- Fat: 5g

- Fiber: 4g

Notes:

- Include a pinch of chili flakes for a hint of heat.

Eggplant and Chickpea Curry

A flavorful and satisfying curry with eggplant, chickpeas, and aromatic flavour.

Prep Time: 15 minutes

Cook Time: 25 minutes

Servings: 4

Ingredients:

- 1 big eggplant, diced

- 1 can chickpeas, drained and washed

- 2 glasses tomato sauce

- 1 container coconut milk

- 1 teaspoon curry powder

- 1 teaspoon turmeric

- 1 teaspoon cumin

- Cooked brown rice (discretionary, for serving)

Instructions:

1. Sauté diced eggplant until softened.

2. Include chickpeas, tomato sauce, coconut milk, curry powder, turmeric, and cumin.

3. Stew until flavors merge and serve over brown rice if craved.

Nutritional Information: (Per serving, without rice)

• Calories: 280

• Protein: 8g

• Carbohydrates: 35g

• Fat: 12g

• Fiber: 10g

Notes:

• Garnish with fresh cilantro or mint before serving.

Spinach and Feta Stuffed Chicken Breast

A delicious and flavorful chicken breast stuffed with fresh spinach and crumbled feta.

- **Prep Time:** 15 minutes
- **Cook Time:** 25 minutes
- **Servings:** 2

Ingredients:

- 2 boneless, skinless chicken breasts

- 2 cups fresh spinach leaves

- 1/2 cup feta cheese, crumbled

- 2 cloves garlic, minced

- Lemon juice

- Olive oil

Instructions:

1. Preheat the oven. Butterfly chicken breasts and stuff with fresh spinach, crumbled feta, minced garlic, and a sprinkle of lemon juice.

2. Heat until chicken is cooked through

Nutritional Information: (Per serving)

- Calories: 320

- Protein: 40g

- Carbohydrates: 4g

- Fat: 16g

- Fiber: 2g

Notes:

- Secure the stuffed chicken breasts with toothpicks before baking.

Cauliflower and Chickpea Tacos

A flavorful and plant-based taco option with broiled cauliflower and seasoned chickpeas.

- **Prep Time:** 20 minutes
- **Cook Time:** 25 minutes
- **Servings:** 4

Ingredients:

- 1 medium cauliflower, cut into florets

- 1 can chickpeas, drained and washed

- 1 teaspoon cumin

- 1 teaspoon paprika

- 1 teaspoon garlic powder

- Corn tortillas

- 1 avocado, sliced

- 1/4 cup cilantro, chopped

Instructions:

1. Broil cauliflower and chickpeas with cumin, paprika, and garlic powder.

2. Fill corn tortillas with the broiled mixture and top with avocado slices and chopped cilantro.

Nutritional Information: (Per serving)

- Calories: 280

- Protein: 8g

- Carbohydrates: 35g

- Fat: 14g

- Fiber: 10g

Note:

- Sprinkle with lime juice for an additional burst of flavour.

Mediterranean Quinoa Bowl

A dynamic and flavorful bowl including quinoa, cherry tomatoes, cucumber, Kalamata olives, red onion, and crumbled feta.

- **Prep Time:** 15 minutes
- **Servings:** 4

Ingredients:

- 2 cups cooked quinoa

- 1 glass cherry tomatoes, halved

- 1 cucumber, diced

- 1/2 container Kalamata olives, sliced

- 1/4 cup red onion, daintily cut

- 1/2 cup feta cheese, crumbled

- Olive oil and balsamic vinegar dressing

Instructions:

1. In a bowl, combine cooked quinoa, cherry tomatoes, cucumber, Kalamata olives, red onion, and crumbled feta cheese.

2. Sprinkle with olive oil and balsamic vinegar dressing and toss gently.

Nutritional Information: (Per serving)

- Calories: 320

- Protein: 12g

- Carbohydrates: 40g

- Fat: 14g

- Fiber: 6g

Notes:

- For a Mediterranean touch dress with fresh basil or oregano

Baked Lemon Herb Salmon

A light and flavorful baked salmon dish with a zesty lemon and herb marinade.

- **Prep Time:** 10 minutes
- **Cook Time:** 15 minutes
- **Servings:** 4

Ingredients:

- 4 salmon fillets

- 1/4 cup fresh lemon juice

- 2 cloves garlic, minced

- 2 tablespoons fresh herbs (parsley, dill, or thyme), chopped

- 2 tablespoons olive oil

Instructions:

1. Preheat the oven and put salmon fillets on a baking sheet.

2. In a bowl, mix lemon juice, minced garlic, chopped herbs, and olive oil to form a marinade.

3. Brush the salmon fillets with the marinade.

4. Bake in the preheated oven for 15 minutes or until the salmon is cooked through.

Nutritional Information: (Per serving)

- Calories: 300

- Protein: 30g

- Carbohydrates: 2g

- Fat: 20g

- Fiber: 0g

Notes:

- Serve with steamed vegetables or a side salad for a complete meal.

Vegetable Stir-Fry with Tofu

A quick and nutritious stir-fry including tofu and an array of colorful vegetables.

- **Prep Time**: 15 minutes
- **Cook Time:** 10 minutes
- **Servings:** 4

Ingredients:

- 1 block tofu, cubed

- 2 glasses broccoli florets

- 1 bell pepper, cut

- 1 container julienned carrots

- 1 glass snap peas

- 1 tablespoon grated ginger

- 3 tablespoons low-sodium soy sauce

Instructions:

1. Sauté tofu, broccoli, bell pepper, carrots, snap peas, and grated ginger in a skillet.

2. Include low-sodium soy sauce and stir-fry until vegetables are tender.

3. Serve over brown rice or quinoa if wanted.

Nutritional Information: (Per serving)

- Calories: 250

- Protein: 15g

- Carbohydrates: 20g

- Fat: 12g

- Fiber: 6g

Notes:

- Feel free to customize with your favorite vegetables and adjust soy sauce to taste.

Turmeric Chickpea Curry

A warming and flavorful chickpea curry infused with turmeric, cumin, and coriander.

- **Prep Time:** 15 minutes
- **Cook Time:** 25 minutes
- **Servings:** 4

Ingredients:

- 2 cans chickpeas, drained and washed

- 1 can coconut milk

- 1 glass tomato sauce

- 1 onion, diced

- 3 cloves garlic, minced

- 1 teaspoon turmeric

- 1 teaspoon cumin

- 1 teaspoon coriander

Instructions:

1. Sauté diced onions and minced garlic until softened.

2. Include chickpeas, coconut milk, tomato sauce, turmeric, cumin, and coriander.

3. Simmer until flavors merge and serve over brown rice or quinoa.

Nutritional Information: (Per serving)

- Calories: 350

- Protein: 12g

- Carbohydrates: 40g

- Fat: 18g

- Fiber: 12g

Notes:

- Garnish with fresh cilantro and serve with a side of naan bread.

Quinoa Stuffed Bell Peppers

Colorful bell peppers stuffed with a tasty blend of quinoa, black beans, corn, and salsa.

- **Prep Time:** 20 minutes
- **Cook Time:** 25 minutes
- **Servings**: 4

Ingredients:

- 2 cups cooked quinoa

- 1 can black beans, drained and washed

- 1 container corn bits

- 1 glass salsa

- 4 bell peppers, halved

- 1 avocado, sliced

Instructions:

1. Mix cooked quinoa, black beans, corn, and salsa in a bowl.

2. Stuff bell peppers with the quinoa mixture.

3. Bake in the oven for 25 minutes or until peppers are soft.

4. Serve with sliced avocado on top.

Nutritional Information: (Per serving)

- Calories: 320

- Protein: 10g

- Carbohydrates: 45g

- Fat: 12g

- Fiber: 10g

Notes:

• Top with a dollop of Greek yogurt or a sprinkle of cheese before serving.

Grilled Chicken and Vegetable Skewers

Tender chicken and dynamic vegetables barbecued to perfection on skewers.

- **Prep Time:** 15 minutes
- **Cook Time:** 15 minutes
- **Servings:** 4

Ingredients:

• 1 pound chicken breast, cubed

• 2 zucchinis, cut

• 1 container cherry tomatoes

• 1 red onion, diced

• 2 tablespoons olive oil

• Fresh herbs (rosemary, thyme)

• Salt and pepper as dresired

Instructions:

1. Marinate chicken cubes in olive oil, fresh herbs, salt, and pepper.

2. Thread chicken, zucchini, cherry tomatoes, and red onion onto skewers.

3. Barbecue until chicken is cooked through and vegetables are soft.

Nutritional Information: (Per serving)

- Calories: 280

- Protein: 25g

- Carbohydrates: 15g

- Fat: 12g

- Fiber: 4g

Notes:

- Serve with a side of quinoa or a light serving of mixed greens.

Cauliflower and Lentil Soup

A comforting soup filled with cauliflower, lentils, and aromatic flavors.

- **Prep Time:** 20 minutes
- **Cook Time**: 6
- **Servings:** 30 minutes

Ingredients:

- 1 medium cauliflower, chopped

- 1 cup lentils, washed

- 2 carrots, diced

- 2 celery stalks, chopped

- 1 onion, diced

- 6 glasses vegetable broth

- 1 teaspoon turmeric

- 1 teaspoon cumin

- 1 teaspoon ginger

Instructions:

1. Sauté onions, carrots, and celery until softened.

2. Include cauliflower, lentils, vegetable broth, turmeric, cumin, and ginger.

3. Simmer until lentils are tender and flavors merge.

Nutritional Information: (Per serving)

- Calories: 220

- Protein: 12g

- Carbohydrates: 40g

- Fat: 2g

- Fiber: 12g

Notes:

- Garnish with a squeeze of lemon juice or a swirl of coconut milk.

Baked Cod with Garlic and Herbs

Flaky cod fillets baked with a garlic and herb topping for a light and flavorful supper.

- **Prep Time:** 10 minutes
- **Cook Time:** 15 minutes
- **Servings:** 4

Ingredients:

- 4 cod fillets

- 4 cloves garlic, minced

- 2 tablespoons fresh herbs (parsley, dill)

- 1 lemon, cut

- 3 tablespoons olive oil

- Salt and pepper as dresired

Instructions:

1. Preheat the oven and place cod fillets on a baking sheet.

2. In a bowl, mix minced garlic, chopped herbs, olive oil, salt, and pepper.

3. Spread the mixture over the cod fillets.

4. Put lemon slices on top and bake until the fish is flaky.

Nutritional Information: (Per serving)

• Calories: 220

• Protein: 30g

• Carbohydrates: 2g

• Fat: 10g

• Fiber: 0g

Notes:

• Dish with side of quinoa or steamed asparagus.

Sweet Potato and Chickpea Curry

A healthy and nutritious curry including sweet potatoes, chickpeas, and aromatic flavors.

- **Prep Time:** 20 minutes
- **Cook Time:** 25 minutes
- **Servings:** 4

Ingredients:

- 2 large sweet potatoes, diced

- 2 cans chickpeas, drained and rinsed

- 1 can coconut milk

- 1 tablespoon curry powder

- 1 teaspoon turmeric

- 1 teaspoon cumin

- 2 cups spinach leaves

Instructions:

1. Sauté sweet potatoes until slightly soft.

2. Include chickpeas, coconut milk, curry powder, turmeric, cumin, and spinach.

3. Simmer until sweet potatoes are completely cooked and spinach is shriveled.

Nutritional Information: (Per serving)

- Calories: 350

- Protein: 10g

- Carbohydrates: 50g

- Fat: 14g

- Fiber: 12g

Notes:

- Serve over brown rice or quinoa for a complete dinner.

Mushroom and Spinach Stuffed Chicken Breast

A flavorful and wholesome dish with chicken breasts stuffed with mushrooms and spinach.

- **Prep Time**: 15 minutes
- **Cook Time**: 25 minutes
- **Servings**: 4

Ingredients:

- 4 boneless, skinless chicken breasts

- 2 glasses mushrooms, chopped

- 2 glasses baby spinach

- 2 cloves garlic, minced

- 2 tablespoons olive oil

- Salt and pepper as desired

Instructions:

1. Preheat the oven and butterfly chicken breasts.

2. Sauté mushrooms, infant spinach, and minced garlic in olive oil until softened.

3. Stuff the chicken breasts with the mushroom and spinach blend.

4. Heat until chicken is cooked through.

5. Serve

Nutritional Information: (Per serving)

- Calories: 300

- Protein: 40g

- Carbohydrates: 4g

- Fat: 14g

- Fiber: 2g

Notes:

- Secure the stuffed chicken breasts with toothpicks before heating.

Zucchini Noodles with Pesto and Cherry Tomatoes

A light and refreshing supper alternative with zucchini noodles tossed in pesto and cherry tomatoes.

- **Prep Time:** 15 minutes
- **Cook Time**: 5 minutes
- **Servings**: 2

Ingredients:

- 4 zucchinis, spiralized into noodles

- 1 container cherry tomatoes, halved

- 1/2 glass pesto sauce

- 2 tablespoons pine nuts (discretionary)

Instructions:

1. Sauté zucchini noodles until soft.

2. Toss with pesto sauce and cherry tomatoes.

3. Top with pine nuts if craved.

Nutritional Information: (Per serving)

• Calories: 250

• Protein: 5g

• Carbohydrates: 15g

• Fat: 20g

• Fiber: 5g

Notes:

• Garnish with fresh basil or grated Parmesan cheese for extra flavor.

These supper recipes are planned to be both tasty and anti-inflammatory. Adjust ingredients and portions based on personal preferences and dietary needs.

Greek Yogurt Parfait with Berries

A refreshing and protein-packed parfait with Greek yogurt, mixed berries, and a touch of honey.

- **Prep Time:** 5 minutes
- **Servings:** 2

Ingredients:

• 1 glass Greek yogurt

• 1 glass blended berries (blueberries, strawberries, raspberries)

• 2 tablespoons honey

• 2 tablespoons almonds (discretionary)

Instructions:

1. In a glass or bowl, layer Greek yogurt with blended berries.

2. Sprinkle nectar over the top and sprinkle with almonds if wanted.

3. Repeat the layers and enjoy!

Nutritional Information: (Per serving)

- Calories: 250

- Protein: 20g

- Carbohydrates: 30g

- Fat: 8g

- Fiber: 5g

Notes:

- Alter sweetness by including more or less honey according to taste.

Turmeric Roasted Chickpeas

Crunchy broiled chickpeas with a hint of turmeric, making a flavorful and satisfying snack.

- **Prep Time:** 5 minutes
- **Cook Time:** 30 minutes
- **Servings:** 4

Ingredients:

- 2 cans chickpeas, drained and washed

- 2 tablespoons olive oil

- 1 teaspoon turmeric

- 1 teaspoon cumin

- 1/2 teaspoon paprika

- Salt and pepper as desired

Instructions:

1. Preheat the oven to 400°F (200°C).

2. In a bowl, toss chickpeas with olive oil, turmeric, cumin, paprika, salt, and pepper.

3. Spread chickpeas on a heating sheet and broil for 30 minutes or until crispy.

4. Permit to cool before serving.

Nutritional Information: (Per serving)

- Calories: 180

- Protein: 8g

- Carbohydrates: 25g

- Fat: 6g

- Fiber: 7g

Notes:

- Test with diverse flavors for varied flavor profiles.

Cucumber Avocado Salsa

A refreshing salsa with diced cucumber, avocado, tomatoes, red onion, lime juice, and cilantro.

- **Prep Time:** 10 minutes
- **Servings:** 4

Ingredients:

- 1 cucumber, diced

- 1 avocado, diced

- 1 container tomatoes, diced

- 1/4 glass red onion, finely chopped

- 2 tablespoons lime juice

- 2 tablespoons cilantro, chopped

Instructions:

1. In a bowl, mix cucumber, avocado, tomatoes, red onion, lime juice, and cilantro.

2. Toss tenderly to combine.

3. Serve with whole grain crackers.

Nutritional Information: (Per serving)

- Calories: 120

- Protein: 2g

- Carbohydrates: 10g

- Fat: 9g

- Fiber: 4g

Notes:

- Add lime juice and cilantro to taste.

Kale Chips

Crispy kale chips prepared with dietary yeast and sea salt for a nutritious and flavorful snack.

- **Prep Time:** 10 minutes
- **Cook Time**: 15 minutes
- **Servings:** 4

Ingredients:

- 1 bunch kale, washed and torn into pieces

- 2 tablespoons olive oil

- 2 tablespoons dietary yeast

- Sea salt as desired

Instructions:

1. Preheat the oven to 350°F (175°C).

2. Massage kale leaves with olive oil, dietary yeast, and sea salt.

3. Spread kale on a baking sheet in a single layer.

4. Bake for 15 minutes or until crisp.

5. Allow to cool before serving.

Nutritional Information: (Per serving)

• Calories: 80

• Protein: 5g

• Carbohydrates: 7g

• Fat: 4g

• Fiber: 3g

Notes:

• Try with different seasonings such as garlic powder or smoked paprika.

Apple Slices with Almond Butter

Slices of fresh apple combined with creamy almond butter for a satisfying and nutrient-rich snack.

- **Prep Time:** 5 minutes
- **Servings:** 2

Ingredients:

- 2 apples, cut

- 4 tablespoons almond butter

Instructions:

1. Cut apples into lean wedges.

2. Dip apple slices into almond butter and enjoy!

Nutritional Information: (Per serving)

- Calories: 250

- Protein: 6g

- Carbohydrates: 30g

- Fat: 15g

- Fiber: 7g

Notes:

- Select your favorite apple variety for extra sweetness or poignancy.

Chia Seed Pudding with Berries

A tasty chia seed pudding made with almond milk, vanilla extract, and topped with mixed berries.

- **Prep Time**: 5 minutes (plus chilling time)
- **Servings**: 2

Ingredients:

- 1/2 glass chia seeds

- 2 glasses almond milk

- 1 teaspoon vanilla extract

- 1 glass mixed berries

- 2 tablespoons maple syrup (discretionary)

Instructions:

1. In a bowl, mix chia seeds, almond milk, and vanilla extract.

2. Refrigerate for at least 2 hours or overnight until a pudding consistency is accomplished.

3. Top with mixed berries and a sprinkle of maple syrup if wanted.

Nutritional Information: (Per serving)

- Calories: 220

- Protein: 8g

- Carbohydrates: 30g

- Fat: 10g

- Fiber: 12g

Notes:

- Alter sweetness with more or less maple syrup.

Trail Mix with Nuts and Seeds

A customizable trail mix including almonds, walnuts, pumpkin seeds, sunflower seeds, dried cranberries, and dark chocolate chips.

- **Prep Time:** 5 minutes
- **Servings:** 4

Ingredients:

- 1/2 container almonds

- 1/2 container walnuts

- 1/4 container pumpkin seeds

- 1/4 cup sunflower seeds

- 1/4 glass dried cranberries or raisins

- 1/4 glass dark chocolate chips

Instructions:

1. Mix all ingredients in a bowl.

2. Portion into little snack sacks for simple on-the-go enjoyment.

Nutritional Information: (Per serving)

- Calories: 250

- Protein: 8g

- Carbohydrates: 15g

- Fat: 18g

• Fiber: 4g

Notes:

• Make your custom mix by including your favorite nuts, seeds, and dried fruits.

Hummus with Veggie Sticks

A classic and nutritious snack including hummus matched with carrot sticks, cucumber cuts, and bell pepper strips.

- **Prep Time:** 10 minutes
- **Servings:** 4

Ingredients:

• 1 cup hummus

• 2 carrots, cut into sticks

• 1 cucumber, cut

• 1 bell pepper, cut into strip

Instructions:

1. Arrange hummus, carrot sticks, cucumber slices, and bell pepper strips on a platter.

2. Dip veggies into hummus and enjoy!

Nutritional Information: (Per serving)

• Calories: 150

• Protein: 6g

• Carbohydrates: 20g

• Fat: 6g

• Fiber: 6g

Notes:

• Select a variety of colorful vegetables for a outwardly engaging snack.

Roasted Edamame

Crispy broiled edamame prepared with garlic powder, smoked paprika, and sea salt.

- **Prep Time:** 5 minutes

- **Cook Time**: 15 minutes

- **Servings**: 4

Ingredients:

- 2 glasses edamame (defrosted if frozen)

- 2 tablespoons olive oil

- 1 teaspoon garlic powder

- 1/2 teaspoon smoked paprika

- Sea salt as desired

Instructions:

1. Preheat the oven to 400°F (200°C).

2. In a bowl, toss edamame with olive oil, garlic powder, smoked paprika, and sea salt.

3. Spread edamame on a baking sheet and broil for 15 minutes or until crispy.

4. Permit to cool before serving.

Nutritional Information: (Per serving)

• Calories: 120

• Protein: 10g

• Carbohydrates: 8g

• Fat: 6g

• Fiber: 4g

Notes:

• Sprinkle with extra sea salt if wanted.

Whole Grain Toast with Avocado

A straightforward and fulfilling nibble highlighting entirety grain toast topped with pounded avocado and cut cherry tomatoes.

- **Prep Time**: 5 minutes
- **Servings**: 2

Ingredients:

• 2 slices whole grain bread, toasted

- 1 avocado, pounded

- 1 glass cherry tomatoes, cut

- Black pepper to taste

Instructions:

1. Toast whole grain bread slices until golden brown.

2. Spread pounded avocado on each slice.

3. Top with sliced cherry tomatoes and sprinkle with black pepper.

Nutritional Information: (Per serving)

- Calories: 220

- Protein: 6g

- Carbohydrates: 30g

- Fat: 10g

- Fiber: 8g

Notes:

- Include a squeeze of lemon juice for additional flavor.

These anti-inflammatory snack recipes are planned to be both tasty and nutritious. Portion sizes should be adjusted to suit personal preferences and dietary requirements.

Berry and Chia Seed Pudding

A nutritious and delicious chia seed pudding infused with the goodness of mixed berries.

- **Prep Time:** 5 minutes (plus chilling time)
- **Servings:** 2

Ingredients:

- 1 glass mixed berries (blueberries, strawberries, raspberries)

- 1/4 glass chia seeds

- 1 1/2 glass almond milk

- 2 tablespoons maple syrup (optional)

Instructions:

1. In a blender, blend mixed berries and almond milk until smooth.

2. In a bowl, mix the berry blend with chia seeds and maple syrup.

3. Refrigerate for at least 2 hours or overnight until the pudding thickens.

4. Serve chilled and enjoy!

Nutritional Information: (Per serving)

- Calories: 180

- Protein: 4g

- Carbohydrates: 25g

- Fat: 8g

- Fiber: 10g

Notes:

- Experiment with different berries for varied flavors.

Turmeric Mango Sorbet

A refreshing fruit juice with the tropical goodness of mango and the anti-inflammatory benefits of turmeric.

- **Prep Time**: 10 minutes (plus freezing time)
- **Servings:** 4

Ingredients:

- 3 cups mango chunks

- 1/2 glass coconut milk

- 1 teaspoon turmeric

- 2 tablespoons honey or agave syrup

Instructions:

1. In a blender, blend mango chunks, coconut milk, turmeric, and honey.

2. Blend until smooth.

3. Pour the mixture into an ice cream maker and stir according to the manufacturer's instructions, or pour into a shallow container and freeze, stirring occasionally.

4. Once set, scoop and serve.

Nutritional Information: (Per serving)

- Calories: 150

- Protein: 2g

- Carbohydrates: 35g

- Fat: 2g

- Fiber: 3g

Notes:

- Adjust sweetness by adding more or less honey.

Dark Chocolate Avocado Mousse

A velvety chocolate mousse made with ripe avocados, offering a rich and guilt-free indulgence.

- **Prep Time:** 15 minutes
- **Servings:** 4

Ingredients:

- 2 ripe avocados

- 1/2 cup dark chocolate (70% cocoa or higher), melted

- 1/4 glass maple syrup

- 1 teaspoon vanilla extract

Instructions:

1. Puree avocados in a food processor until smooth.

2. Add melted dark chocolate, maple syrup, and vanilla extract.

3. Blend until well mixed.

4. Refrigerate for at least 1 hour before serving.

5. Serve into serving dishes and enjoy!

Nutritional Information: (Per serving)

- Calories: 220

- Protein: 3g

- Carbohydrates: 22g

- Fat: 15g

- Fiber: 6g

Notes:

- Garnish with berries or a sprinkle of cocoa powder if desired.

Baked Cinnamon Apples

Warm and comforting baked apples with a topping of cinnamon and a crunchy walnut.

- **Prep Time:** 10 minutes
- **Cook Time:** 25 minutes
- **Servings:** 4

Ingredients:

- 4 apples, sliced

- 1 teaspoon cinnamon

- 1/2 teaspoon nutmeg

- 1/2 cup walnuts, chopped

Instructions:

1. Preheat the oven to 375°F (190°C).

2. In a bowl, s apple slices with cinnamon and nutmeg.

3. Arrange apples in a baking dish and sprinkle with chopped walnuts.

4. Bake for 25 minutes or until apples are soft.

5. Serve warm and enjoy!

Nutritional Information: (Per serving)

• Calories: 180

• Protein: 2g

• Carbohydrates: 30g

• Fat: 8g

• Fiber: 6g

Notes:

• Top with a dollop of Greek yogurt for extra creaminess.

Coconut and Berry Popsicles

Cooling popsicles with coconut milk and mixed berries, perfect for a refreshing treat.

• **Prep Time:** 10 minutes (plus freezing time)

- **Servings:** 6

Ingredients:

- 1 can (14 oz) coconut milk

- 1 cup berries mixture (blueberries, strawberries, raspberries)

- 2 tablespoons shredded coconut

- 2 tablespoons honey or agave syrup

Instructions:

1. In a blender, add coconut milk, mixed berries, shredded coconut, and honey.

2. Blend until smooth.

3. Pour the mixture into popsicle molds and freeze until solid.

4. Run molds under warm water to release popsicles and enjoy!

Nutritional Information: (Per serving)

- Calories: 120

- Protein: 1g

- Carbohydrates: 10g

- Fat: 8g

- Fiber: 2g

Notes:

- Experiment with different berries or add a squeeze of lime juice for extra zing.

Turmeric Golden Milk Ice Cream

A soothing and creamy ice cream with the warm flavors of turmeric and ginger.

- **Prep Time:** 15 minutes (plus freezing time)
- **Servings:** 6

Ingredients:

- 2 cans full-fat coconut milk

- 1 1/2 teaspoons turmeric

- 1 teaspoon ginger

- 1/2 cup maple syrup

Instructions:

1. In a bowl, mix together coconut milk, turmeric, ginger, and maple syrup.

2. Stir in an ice cream maker according to the manufacturer's instructions or pour into a shallow container and freeze, stir occasionally.

3. Once set, scoop and serve.

Nutritional Information: (Per serving)

- Calories: 220

- Protein: 1g

- Carbohydrates: 25g

- Fat: 14g

- Fiber: 0g

Notes:

- Sprinkle with a pinch of black pepper for an extra kick.

A refreshing frozen fresh fruit juice with tropical pineapple and a hint of mint for a burst of flavor.

Prep Time: 10 minutes (plus freezing time)

Servings: 4

Ingredients:

- 3 cups fresh pineapple chunks

- 1/4 cup fresh mint leaves

- 2 tablespoons lime juice

- 3 tablespoons agave syrup

Instructions:

1. In a blender, add pineapple chunks, mint leaves, lime juice, and agave syrup.

2. Blend until smooth.

3. Pour the mixture into an ice cream maker and stir according to the manufacturer's instructions, or freeze in a shallow container, stirring occasionally.

4. Once set, scoop and serve.

Nutritional Information: (Per serving)

- Calories: 110

- Protein: 1g

- Carbohydrates: 30g

- Fat: 0g

- Fiber: 2g

Notes:

- Garnish with a sprig of fresh mint for a decorative touch.

Walnut and Date Energy Bites

A quick and energy-boosting snack featuring the natural sweetness of dates and the crunch of walnuts.

- **Prep Time**: 15 minutes
- **Servings:** 12

Ingredients:

- 1 cup walnuts

- 1 cup pitted dates

- 2 tablespoons chia seeds

- 1 teaspoon vanilla extract

Instructions:

1. In a food processor, blend walnuts, dates, chia seeds, and vanilla extract until a dough forms.

2. Roll the mixture into small energy bites.

3. Place in the refrigerator for at least 30 minutes before serving.

4. Enjoy these nutritious bites!

Nutritional Information: (Per serving - 2 bites)

- Calories: 120

- Protein: 2g

- Carbohydrates: 15g

- Fat: 6g

- Fiber: 3g

Notes:

- Add a pinch of sea salt for a sweet-savory flavor.

Blueberry Almond Crisp

A delicious blueberry almond crisp with a crumbly topping, serving as a healthier alternative to traditional desserts.

Prep Time: 15 minutes

Cook Time: 30 minutes

Servings: 6

Ingredients:

- 4 cups fresh or frozen blueberries

- 1 cup almond flour

- 1 cup rolled oats

- 1/4 cup maple syrup

Instructions:

1. Preheat the oven to 350°F (175°C).

2. In a bowl, mix blueberries with almond flour and rolled oats.

3. Drizzle maple syrup over the mixture and mix until combined.

4. Transfer the mixture to a baking dish and bake for 30 minutes or until the top is golden brown.

5. Allow to cool slightly before serving.

Nutritional Information: (Per serving)

• Calories: 240

• Protein: 5g

• Carbohydrates: 35g

• Fat: 10g

• Fiber: 6g

Notes:

• Serve with a spoonful of Greek yogurt or a scoop of vanilla ice cream.

Lemon Ginger Turmeric Cookies

Zesty and spiced cookies featuring almond flour, coconut oil, and the anti-inflammatory benefits of turmeric and ginger.

- **Prep Time:** 10 minutes
- **Cook Time**: 12 minutes
- **Servings**: 18 cookies

Ingredients:

- 2 cups almond flour

- 1/4 cup coconut oil, melted

- 1/4 cup maple syrup

- Zest of 1 lemon

- 1 teaspoon ground ginger

- 1 teaspoon turmeric

Instructions:

1. Preheat the oven to 350°F (175°C).

2. In a bowl, mix almond flour, melted coconut oil, maple syrup, lemon zest, ground ginger, and turmeric until a dough forms.

3. Scoop tablespoon-sized portions onto a baking sheet.

4. Use the back of a fork to flatten each cookie

5. Bake for 12 minutes or until the sides are golden.

6. Allow to cool before serving.

Nutritional Information: (Per serving - 1 cookie)

• Calories: 100

• Protein: 3g

• Carbohydrates: 7g

• Fat: 7g

• Fiber: 1g

Notes:

• Experiment with different citrus zests for unique flavor combinations.

CONCLUSION

As we conclude our journey through the "Anti-Inflammatory Diet Cookbook for Beginners: The Complete Culinary Guide to Reducing Inflammation and Healing the Immune System for Whole Body Wellness with Easy, Delicious, and Healthy Recipes," it is critical to emphasize the profound importance of living an anti-inflammatory lifestyle. This comprehensive book has offered not just a collection of recipes, but also a road map to holistic well-being, highlighting the importance of our food choices in relation to our entire health.

Recap of the Importance of an Anti-Inflammatory Diet

As we reflect the content on these pages, it becomes clear that the anti-inflammatory diet is significantly more than just a collection of nutrients. It is an effective tool for reducing chronic inflammation, supporting the immune system, and boosting overall wellbeing. The carefully picked recipes offered here leverage the power of nutrient-dense foods high in antioxidants and essential fatty acids—key components in the fight against inflammation. The emphasis on embracing various, bright foods demonstrates the lifestyle's adaptability and accessibility, allowing anybody, regardless of dietary preferences, to begin on this transforming journey.

Encouragement for Beginners to Continue Their Journey toward Whole-Body Wellness

A warm congratulations to the beginners who have begun on this fascinating trip. Embracing a new way of eating might be a daunting task, but the benefits are plentiful and lasting. The first actions you've made toward an anti-inflammatory lifestyle are more than just a dietary shift; they represent a commitment to your well-being. Continue to enjoy the aromas of nutritious meals, cherish the newfound energy, and celebrate the steady improvements in your general health. Remember that this is a journey, not a race, and that every healthy choice contributes to the tremendous transformation taking place within.

Invitation to Explore the Diverse and Delicious World
of Anti-Inflammatory Cooking for Long-Term Health
Benefits

This culinary tour finishes with an open invitation to explore the wide and wonderful world of anti-inflammatory cuisine. The recipes shown here are only a sample of the numerous options that this lifestyle provides. Experiment with herbs and spices, look into seasonal food, and experience the thrill of creating meals that not only satisfy the taste senses but also nourish the body from inside. The anti-inflammatory journey is more than simply a temporary change; it is a lifetime commitment to bright health and longevity.

In essence, this cookbook serves as a compass, guiding you toward a life in which your food choices are a source of healing and energy. The path to reduced inflammation, improved immune function, and overall wellbeing is a never-ending, rewarding adventure. So, keep savoring the tastes, enjoying the trip, and embracing the wonderful transformation that occurs when you fuel your body with

the nutritious, anti-inflammatory goodness it requires.
Bon appétit to a life well lived!

www.ingramcontent.com/pod-product-compliance
Lightning Source LLC
Chambersburg PA
CBHW061932270726
48660CB00004BA/1557